Eat More to Lose Weight—Not Less!

Eat More to Lose Weight–Not Less!

Table Of Contents

Foreword

Chapter 1:
Introduction

Chapter 2:
Healthy Eating Habits Tips

Chapter 3:
Food Quantities and Weight Loss

Chapter 4:
A Balanced Diet In Weight Loss

Chapter 5:
The Blood Type Principle of Weight Loss

Chapter 6:
The Science of Weight Loss

Chapter 7:
The Magic Bullet of Protein

Chapter 8:
Meal Timing

Chapter 9:
Calorie Counting Is Dead

Wrapping Up
Benefits Of Right Food To Health

Foreword

The first chapter of this course is focused on how changing lifestyle – more healthful diets and more exercises - helps you to lose weight and gain good health, and why starving yourself to lose weight is unnecessary and even dangerous. Chapters 9 to 10 are about healthy eating habits, food combinations and quantities that promotes weight loss, the science of losing weight, contribution of protein to getting fit, timing your meals, and the health benefits of eating the right foods. Get all the info you need here.

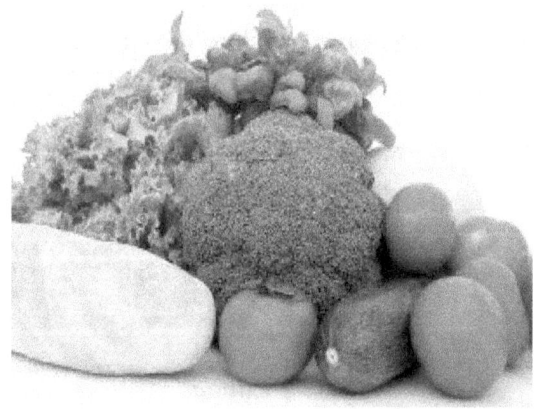

Eat More, Not Less To Lose Weight!
Build Your Health And Your Body By Eating Right, Not Less!

Chapter 1:
Introduction

Synopsis

This course teaches you how to lose weight without the customary calorie counting that is often the basis of most weight loss diets. To be sure, low-calorie diets are too fast but it is a well known fact that they pose special hardships and gains are hard to sustain. Composed of 10 chapters, this course provides you with greater understanding of the needs of your body and how this knowledge help you follow a diet that induces weight loss and sustains your gains without effort.

Weight loss should result in a healthier you, not just a slimmer you. There are a variety of methods that try to make you believe you can solve your weight issues easily and fast. There are miracle diet pills and diets that drastically reduce your calorie and your general food consumption levels promising rapid weight reduction, which in the end leave you grappling with tremendous hunger pangs and dangerous side effects.

Losing Weight Naturally

There are no such things as miracle treatments for a weight loss problem. Of course, it is possible to become slim through the use of fad diets, but you will not be healthy because crash diets deny you nutrients that are necessary for your body to function properly.

It weakens your health and what's more you are likely to go back to your former eating habits since the fad diet taught you nothing. You will be having the same problem again and again. Worse, according to studies people who have undergone repetitive weight loss diets, then became permanently overweight, and are in worse health than those who hadn't tried solving their weight problems at all.

Change Your Lifestyle

Changing your lifestyle is actually the most effective way of losing weight and staying healthy. A switch from a calorie-loaded diet to a low calorie diet is a must. You do not actually have to reduce food intake, just eat healthful foods - more vegetables and fruits, lean meats, whole grains and others.

Regular exercise should also help you lose weight as well as maintaining good health. Since you are taking in fewer calories from your diet, your workouts should be burning fat deposits in your body.

The workouts may not be even programmed. Sports and games like tennis or basketball are excellent exercise and if you feel like other forms of exercise are a chore. You can actually enjoy the games though, especially when you play with friends, which means turning exercise into a habit will not be difficult.

The process of getting you down to your appropriate weight through the natural method may be slow, but you feel good the whole time and maintaining gains does not require doing anything outside of your established daily routine.

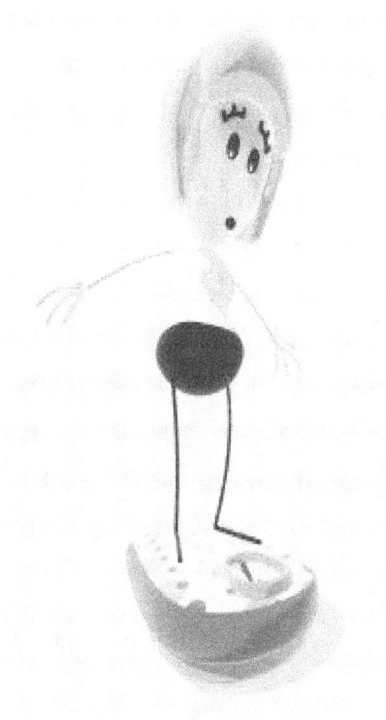

Chapter 2:

Healthy Eating Habit Tips

Synopsis

In a world where fast food is considered a real meal, no wonder there are so many people in a bad shape. The rate of obese people is a cause for alarm but this can all change if everyone gets educated on healthy eating habits.

The secret to healthy eating is all about balance. It's having all the right nutrients, vitamins and calories in one meal. There's really no need to deprive yourself from food that you like. It's about having all of these foods, but in moderation. Like the old saying goes, Too much of anything is bad. This can be applied greatly to the food you eat.

The truth is, what you consume everyday greatly affects your whole attitude and energy level for the whole day. Sure it is convenient but there's so much more to life than a cheeseburger meal or Chinese food take out. It's tasty and you can't help craving it, but experimenting in your kitchen can easily result in the best meal of your life.

So here are some tips for healthy eating habits for a better you:

One Step at a Time

If you are just starting to change into a healthier lifestyle, then do it slowly. Your body has been accustomed to old ways and if you change drastically, it is likely that you will also give up easily.

Eat At Home

Whenever you eat out, you do not have any control on the portions that you will have. You might end up eating more than you need to.

Stop Counting the Calories

Do not be obsessed about that. Instead, look at food in terms of color and freshness. Greens are always good. Colorful fruits are also great for a person's body. These are the food that your body needs more of. So do not feel afraid to eat more of these.

Do Not Skip Meals

If your goal is to lose weight, then it is much better to eat small portions of food 5- 6 times a day. Skipping meals will only retain the fat in your body and may result in overeating.

Snack Healthy

When you're feeling hungry, instead of reaching out for the cupcake, grab that carrot stick instead. Some good examples of food to snack on are fruits, nuts, raisins, cranberries, whole grain crackers, etc.

Enjoy Your Meal

Do not rush the eating process. Take your time and chew your food slowly. When you're already feeling full, then stop eating. Listen to what your body tells you.

Remember To Drink a Lot of Water

Sometimes people confuse thirst with hunger and eat when all they needed was just a glass of water. Drinking water is also good for cleansing the body from toxins and helps in having better digestion.

Along with these tips, you should always remember to have not just good eating habits but also a healthy lifestyle. This means making an effort to exercise regularly. If you are a smoker, then consider quitting and lastly, drink alcoholic beverages moderately.

Chapter 3:
Food Quantities and Weight Loss

Synopsis

When trying to lose weight, dieters tend to focus on the quantity of the food they intake. If you are one of these people wanting to shed pounds, listen up. Here's something that you need to keep in mind:

CHOOSE QUALITY OVER QUANTITY ALL THE TIME.

Most people on a diet tend to drastically cut down on food. Some even starve themselves thinking if they do not eat food, they won't gain weight. Sure, that is true. However, it will also not help you lose weight. In fact, if you stop eating, your body will work on keeping your fats so that you can have the energy you need during the day.

So what does a person have to do? What is the right quantity of food to eat during a diet? How often can a person eat? All of these questions will be answered in this article, so continue reading on.

Small Portions Several Times throughout the Day

Most experts say that there are many more benefits when it comes to losing weight if you eat 5-6 meals per day compared to 3 meals. Granted the meals are small, of course. The reason for this is because your body will have balanced levels of sugar in the blood. Meaning, you won't be feeling intense hunger. When a person is hungry, they tend to eat more than usual.

Eating smaller portions throughout the day will also reduce cholesterol. In studies done by experts, it was proven that having smaller meals consumed 6 times a day decreased cholesterol levels by 5 percent.

Fill that Plate Up With the Right Kind of Stuff

What a person eats greatly affects their weight loss or weight gain. This is why dietitians encourage people to go for quality over quantity. A good example is you might have eaten only crackers for lunch today but also had a huge jug of sweetened drinks. Then that sweetened drink is the culprit when it comes to your weight gain.

If you had a large bowl of fresh salad and water, then that would have been considered a better meal on a diet than the crackers with a sweetened drink. It is much better for the body to take foods that are less in carbohydrates. Taking away bread, pasta, rice or potatoes and replacing it with vegetables will definitely help cut back on fat.

If you are the type of person who will feel full only if you see large portions of food on your plate, then the solution is to fill your plate with the right kind of food. Think colorful fruits and vegetables. Deep colors means higher content of vitamins, minerals and antioxidants. All of these is what your body needs every day.

To commit to a long-term diet, it is important to **like what you eat**. If you hate the thought of just eating vegetables or fruits all day, then do some research on diet recipes. Eating meat is encouraged, so don't cut back on that. As long as it is not always deep fried, then it's still good.

It's really important to enjoy the process. Otherwise, you will easily go back to your old routine. Just remember, too much of anything is bad. Keep everything well balanced and eat only when your body is telling you it's hungry.

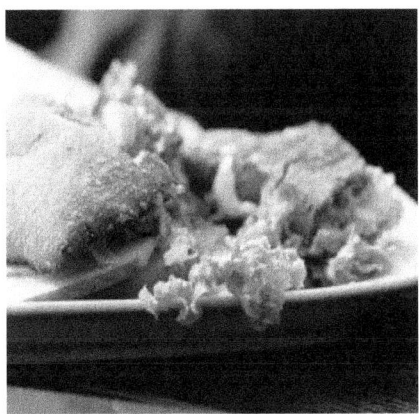

Chapter 4:

A Balanced Diet in Weight Loss

Synopsis

If you have noticed, just a quick search of weight loss on the Internet will immediately provide you with weight loss products like diet pills, weight loss programs and even gym memberships. These can cost a great deal of money and most of them are not even effective. So why not go back to basics and do the easiest and the cheapest thing you can do to lose weight: adopt a balanced diet.

Achieving a balanced diet includes eating the right kind and amount of food that will give you enough nutrients to sustain weight loss. Ideally, your diet should be heavier in fruits and vegetables, whole carbohydrates and low in dietary fats.

Additionally, lean proteins, and lots of water for hydration and exercise are important. Even though we all have different nutrient needs and metabolisms, all these factors are still important to achieve weightloss in the safest and cheapest way.

The Benefits of a Balanced Diet

Opting for a balanced diet to maintain a healthy weight is important in order to achieve weight loss since you are still supplying your body the right amount of vitamins and minerals it needs to function properly. When combined with consistent exercise, it is inevitable that you will lose weight without risking any health problems.

Maintaining a balanced diet with the aim of losing weight is beneficial as compared to products that promise a quick and easy way to weight loss. First, it lessens the risk of your developing cardiovascular diseases like heart diseases and diabetes. It can also aid you in controling these conditions if ever you are suffering from one. This healthy regimen also promotes regular metabolism and a healthy digestive system, which will enable you to lose bad fats and absorb the good ones.

Aside from that, the choice of eating a balanced diet will definitely boost your confidence knowing that you will achieve your desired weight in the healthiest way possible.

How to Start Right

Starting out can be quite a challenge but it should be easy. Always remember the basics of eating more whole-carbohydrates by avoiding foods like chocolates, ice creams, chips, sodas, cookies, cakes and many others. These types of foods contain high amounts of sugar, cholesterol, salt and other unwanted substances.

These foods are also called 'empty calories' since they do not provide nutrients other than calories. Choose to drink fresh fruit juice instead of sodas, as they add approximately 500 calories more to your diet.

With that in mind, plan your meal correctly by adding more of the good kinds of food. You can have a high-fiber cereal with low-fat milk at breakfast, and then lunch would be a grilled turkey sandwich over whole wheat bread and a vegetable salad. Dinner can be baked fish and vegetables.

These are just a few of the simple dishes you can make and they are even easier to prepare. Just keep in mind that every meal should contain a variety of foods, such as fruits, lean proteins, vegetables and high-fiber carbohydrates.

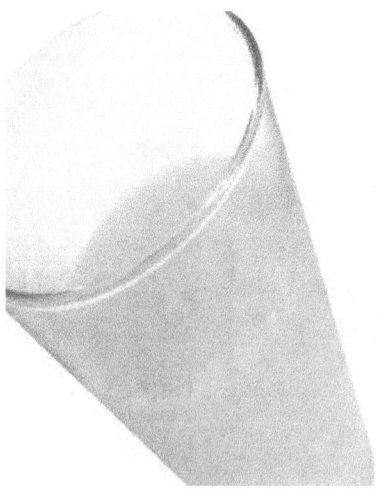

Chapter 5:
The Blood Type Principles of Weight Loss

Synopsis

A lot of people are now understanding the importance of having a healthy body. This is why there is a surge in the health and fitness industry. A lot more people are now going to the gym to try different forms of exercise to get in shape.

People are also trying different kinds of diets, from Atkins to Paleo to South Beach to Weight Watchers. All of these are effective, though some more than others. But did you know that there's a diet that is designed for your blood type? If you have tried almost all of the famous diet trends available and have not seen a lot of results, then this might be the perfect one for you.

This diet was designed by Doctor Peter D'Amado and is called The Blood Group Diet. This new diet is gaining more popularity because a lot of the big names in Hollywood say it's the reason for their amazing bodies. Actors like Courtney Cox and Cheryl Cole swear by it.

So what exactly is The Blood Group Diet and how does it work?

It is believed that each blood group reacts differently to each food. So if you follow the diet designed for you, the chances of losing weight will be higher because your body will absorb food more efficiently.

Let's look at the diet closely. If you have **Blood Type O**, which is the most common blood type in humans, then the diet should be similar to Paleo where it is encouraged to eat more like "hunter-gatherer" style. This means eating food that was available to our ancestors before agriculture growth and advancement in technology happened. High protein and low in carbohydrates is the way to go.

Along with this diet, blood type O people should also do a lot of high intensity cardio like running to complement the diet.

Blood Type A diet is almost the opposite of the diet suggested to Blood Type O. Meaning, their bodies are much more accepting to the more "modern" food. A vegan diet is encouraged, so this means lots of vegetables and carbohydrates like rice, pasta and cereals. However, meat and dairy products such as milk, cheese or butter should be avoided. Meat should be taken in very little quantity.

Blood type A diet is best done with slow and relaxing exercise such as yoga or Pilates.

Blood Type AB can be defined as the most lenient diet. This rare blood type works well with almost every food but with moderation. They have a good immune system, which means they can handle dairy, meat and carbs well. However, vegetables are the most encouraged food to eat. The rest should be eaten in little portions.

When it comes to exercises, Blood type AB should combine both calming and high intensity workouts.

Blood Type B has the least restrictions. Vegetables, fruits, meat, dairy, seafood, rice - these can all be taken as long as it's part of a balanced diet and not taken in big quantities. The only food to avoid are processed foods such as the ones that can be bought in a can (luncheon meat, hotdog, ham etc)

Any activity that involves exercising the brain such as tennis, golf, hiking is the best form of exercise for this blood type.

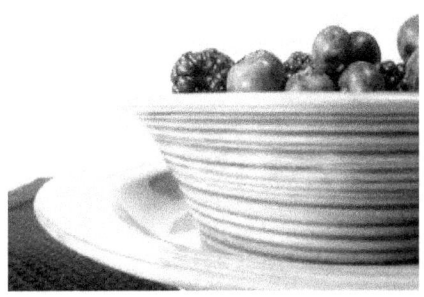

Chapter 6:
The Science of Weight Loss

Synopsis

Weight loss can sometimes be tiring. After thousands of dollars spent on diet programs with all efforts to cut-down calories, it seems that you are not losing weight as you expect it.

Of course, you will then have to check with your doctor or nutritionist to see why you are not losing that much weight and you will end up with 'the look' that strikes the paranoia out of you.

These are just few of the challenges you may encounter when you are into weight loss programs. It can get the best out of you depending on how you take all the challenges up. Well, there is a better way to actually achieve weight loss with 3 easy reminders.

The Science

1. There Is Such A Thing Called 'Real Carbohydrates'

The first thing you need to do is to identify your carbohydrate intake. All of us know that carbohydrates are the main source of energy as carbs are readily converted to glucose, the main substance that is used for energy production. All the excess carbohydrates are turned into fat when they aren't used as energy. Now, what you need to remember is that you need to consume 'real carbohydrates' by choosing foods that are not processed. Replace the processed carbohydrates with natural ones like vegetables and fruits in every meal. Momentarily avoid other carbohydrates like chips, breads, pasta, fast food meals and others.

2. Have you ever heard of high-biological proteins? Choose them among others.

High-biological proteins are what you can think of as complete proteins. They are called such because they contain complete amino acids to provide efficient functions in terms of repairing body tissues and supplying proteins to every muscle in your body. Amino acids work like a team: when one is missing, they cannot function well. So it is good to invest in high-biological proteins by eating natural and grass-fed meats and produce. This includes turkey, beef, chicken, lamb, pork and other animal proteins.

3. There are healthy fats, of course.

If you think that fats are the only culprits of weight gain, you are definitely wrong. Your body also needs fats in order to function well as these substances contribute to temperature control, metabolism regulation and lubrication of vein and arteries. So, have a moderate intake of healthy fats, including avocadoes, coconut oil, olive oil, nuts, olives, seeds and butter. Just remember to consume about 2-3 teaspoons of these fats at every meal.

These are the **three easy steps** that you can always remember for you to have a significant weight loss. Start on these rules and you are off to a good start. It is good to remember that metabolism is as complex as our brain, so the notion of calorie counting does not really apply to all.

The basis of a healthy weight should come from consuming the right amount and kinds of food or to simply put it: the right balance of food. So start your meal right today by investing more on real carbohydrates, high-biological proteins and healthy fats.

Chapter 7:
The Magic Bullet of Protein

Synopsis

When you have just trained so intensely, especially after resting for a while, then you are more prone to get sore muscles a day after your training. Muscle soreness can be very burdensome, as you experience pain in every move you make. With that, you should know all the reasons behind sore muscles and what you can do to prevent them. Well, the basis of this is the consumption of proteins.

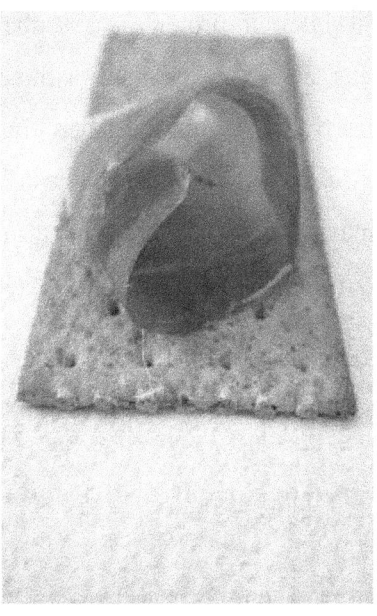

The Essence of Protein to Muscles

Proteins are essential to help tissues repair themselves and supply a leaner body structure. There are so many uses of proteins you may never know. In fact, they can also be used as energy when the carbohydrate sources are empty. Aside from that, they strengthen your immune system and give you skin that is smooth in texture. It has anti-aging benefits, enhances memory and so much more. This is why proteins are pretty valuable and should be saved for their functions instead of using them as energy.

The Right Kind of Proteins

Choosing the right kind of protein is essential to give you the advantage of having a lean body mass without the risk of sore muscles. The advice below is from an expert trainer, Taoist master Tommy Kirchhoff. He studied the popular martial arts Sheng Long Fu and is the Grandmaster of Victor Sheng Long Fu. He is a versatile fitness expert and is credited for contributing effective advice to fitness enthusiasts.

Not all have known this fact: **proteins are made to function equally as compared to carbohydrates and fats.**

So people are so wrong when they just invest in eating chicken alone. All proteins are a definite cure for intense training and they should be eaten in the most absorbable form.

Why?

This is because muscles need an immediate source of protein to supply their needs, especially during a heavy workout. With that, you need to opt for protein powders, as they give the quickest and most absorbable type of proteins to work and repair your body tissues. In order to find out which powdered proteins are best for you, just visit your personal trainer or sports nutritionist. You can also visit a sports house in your area or GNC stores.

Now, if you don't just have the right budget to buy these powdered proteins, which can be expensive by the way, you can opt for egg whites. The only thing that you should remember is this: you have to eat them raw and fresh.

Yes, you can get the most amino acids in raw fresh eggs as compared to cooking them. The reason for this is because as soon as you cook the egg, the structure of its proteins changes significantly, making it less absorbable. So manipulating an egg white, even if you shake, blend or stir them has effects that you may never know. In fact, your body may not even use the proteins completely.

Therefore, whenever you need the best proteins next to the powdered ones, get fresh eggs, separate the yolks (since they contain too much fat and cholesterol) and swallow them up.

Chapter 8:

Meal Timing

Synopsis

Meal timing is an essential part of a balanced diet. When we want to be on the top of our shapely figure, the right kind, amount and timing is important to balance your calories throughout the day. With that, there is no need to restrict yourself from eating lesser foods or depriving your body with the needed ingredients it should use for a day's work.

Our metabolism is different like our identity. Every individual has a different health and lifestyle profile which explains why it is hard to follow a single diet program.

A diet plan may be effective for you, but not for your friend. Even the intensity and duration of exercise may not be suitable for your friend as compared to yours. So to better understand what is actually happening inside your body, here is a basic explanation.

Timing

Breakfast Time:

- The body has fasted from sleep so there is no food intake for 8-12 hours.
- With this occurrence, the energy reserves (in the form of glycogen) are definitely low.
- This is where our muscles are in a state called mild catabolic, since the energy reserves are used for energy while there is no food intake for 8-12 hours.
- The fat stores are being used up as energy. Thus, it is being burned and mobilized.

Your metabolic goal at this time is to replenish the glycogen stores that were used from the fasting hours. You also need to stop your muscles from catabolism so that you will not acquire a state of muscle wasting. Along with that, you also need to support the continuous metabolism of fat.

To do that, you need to have a combination of high quality proteins that are absorbable enough to quickly replenish your muscles from fasting, like eggs and lean meats. You can also mix simple with complex carbohydrates to quickly replenish energy and at the same time, gradually release some of it as you go along your daily routine.

Fat is also important, so make sure to consume essential fatty acids. With that, you can eat walnuts, seeds and avocadoes. You can also make use of little amount of oil like canola oil or flax seed oil.

AM Snack

- The level of your glucose is already gradually balancing out
- The feeling of hunger is increased

Your metabolic goal: give your muscles the strength they need by consuming proteins and enough carbohydrates. It is good to further balance out your glucose level and at the same time, replenish protein stores.

To do that: You need to mix proteins and carbohydrates just enough to attain your metabolic goal. Consider foods with low-glycemic index and you can drink protein shakes, whey proteins from milk and fresh egg whites.

Lunch Time

- The morning snack that you have eaten is burned as energy and you may need more for a full day's work.

Your metabolic goal is to provide your muscles with sufficient calories with carbohydrates and proteins. Lunch can be your largest meal as compared to breakfast and dinner since you will work more after.

To do this, simply mix high-protein meat products like beef or chicken, then opt for high-fiber and low-glycemic carbohydrates. It is also good to invest in essential fatty acids.

PM Snack

- The levels of the glucose in your body are now deteriorating.
- With a few hours of mild fasting, your muscle is in a metabolic state again.

At this time, your metabolic goal is to gradually level your glucose up and stop the muscles from being catabolized.

To do this: Simply choose a snack that is enough to keep you replenished until dinner. Eat proteins that are slowly absorbed like cooked eggs. As for the carbohydrates, choose the ones that are low in sugar but are dense in calories.

Dinner Time

- Your muscles are anabolic as they prepare for another 8-12 hours of fasting during a sleep. This is up until about 12 in the morning.

Your metabolic goals should support your muscles while they are in an anabolic stage so the catabolic state will not impose any health problems in the long run.

With that, you need to eat types of foods that are low in calories but rich in protein. Choose proteins that are slowly absorbed like beef, pork and chicken. Invest in high-fiber carbohydrates and essential fatty acids.

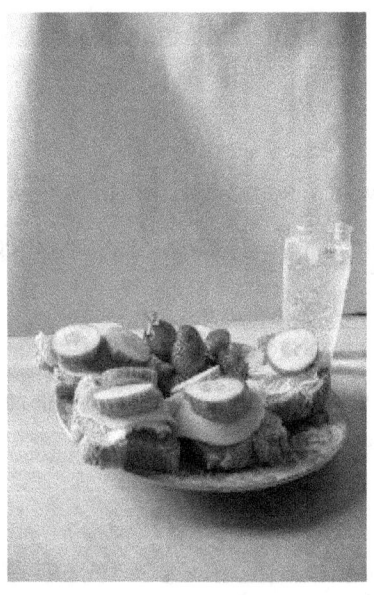

Chapter 9:
Calorie Counting is Dead

Synopsis

Right now, if reports from health agencies are accurate, there could be a billion people in the planet experiencing weight problems. The health and fitness industry which generates billions of dollars in health related revenues continues to churn out various weight loss programs based on drastically reduced calorie diets along with strenuous workouts, and you wonder why the obesity rates are still increasing and whether such an approach is really effective.

Many of the makers of these programs, of course, stress that in order for them to work you heed to persevere, be disciplined and have the tenacity to persist in the face of difficulties that said programs are liable to bring in.

Perhaps the difficulties that you have to undergo when employing these weight loss routines is the main problem which means that all along makers may have been selling an approach that hardly works in the first place. Lose weight fast? You or anyone else for that matter will have a hard time resisting that kind of marketing pitch.

Calorie Deficit, a New and More Effective Approach

Fortunately, some weight loss advocates are trying to shift approaches, from low-calorie diets to less stressful methods. And they base the shift on something that's simple and logical – calorie deficit.

When you are overweight, it only means one thing; you have fat deposits in your body that your metabolism can't process. The question is why your metabolism can't do that. The answer is you are taking more calories than your metabolism can handle. Does this mean that you have to starve yourself in order to lose weight? Of course not, you will be risking your health if you do that and you will end up dealing with worse problems than before.

The key to losing weight without experiencing a whole range of issues is to create a calorie deficit, which simply means that you eat fewer calories than your body demands. Fewer calories are the keywords, not zero-calories. When you take in fewer calories and you work out, your body starts burning your fat deposits to supply you with the energy you need for the workouts. Naturally when your body burns fat deposits every day you will not be far away from your ideal weight.

Advantages

The calorie deficit approach has many advantages that are not present in drastically reduced weight loss diets. You do not need specially prepared meals to ensure the required calorie intake levels. All you need to is to eliminate some of the calorie loaded foods you are in the habit of eating. Your body won't be deprived of energy which allows it to function normally and you wil feel good as you lose weight.

Aside from reducing the calories, your diet has to be as nutritionally balanced as you can make it. You want the natural body cleansers in it to help your metabolism work more efficiently. You need the proteins and other nutrients that promote good health.

Benefits

One of the benefits of the calorie deficit approach to losing weight is your health is never compromised; instead, you can become healthier. And unlike low calorie diets that make it difficult for you to protect gains because the deprivation will make the foods you used to eat hard to resist, with this approach since its slower the diet will be a habit by the time you have realized your weight reduction goals.

Wrapping Up
Benefits of Right Food to Health

By now you should fully understand that healthy eating is not synonymous at all to dieting – and especially where dangerous fad diets are concerned. Eating the right food may be a struggle at the start, but it's a challenge that's guaranteed to promise numerous health benefits once healthy eating becomes a regular part of your life.

A Balanced Intake of Vitamins, Minerals, and Other Nutrients

By knowing which foods to eat more of and which ones to eat in moderation, you will be able to benefit from a balanced intake of vitamins, minerals, and essential nutrients. This may come as a surprise to you, but too much of any particular vitamin can actually be detrimental to your health.

Vitamin D toxicity, for instance, can lead to excess content of calcium in your body, which could be bad for your bones and heart. On the other hand, vitamin deficiencies are – as you know – just as bad. Hypocobalaminemia or Vitamin B12 deficiency can inflict long-term damage on nerve tissues if the disorder is not addressed and left untreated.

Higher Energy Levels

A lot of people have a hard time understanding the importance of energy because it's something you can't actually see. Even so, energy is something that will make a difference in how you feel especially as you advance in years. Higher energy levels allow you to be more physically active – especially compared to peers who haven't yet appreciated the benefits of healthy eating. You get to enjoy a better overall quality of life as well as spend a more productive time not just at work but when you spend time with your loved ones as well.

Stress Reduction or Elimination

People may not directly die of stress, but you can be sure that stress is one of the leading contributing causes to diseases that do kill. Stress doesn't just affect your health. It can also affect your career and personal relationships. Even the way you interact with your family may be negatively affected if you let stress get the better of you.
Thankfully, healthy eating is one of the best ways to combat stress. It puts you in a better mood and makes you less vulnerable to anxiety and depression.

Lower Blood Pressure

Hypertension is the other name for high blood pressure and is a symptom for many different types of chronic diseases. Most of those diseases affect your heart and may have life-threatening consequences. Maintenance for hypertension can be quite expensive and surgery for critical cases is even more cost-prohibitive. You can avoid all such headaches in the future, however, if you simply opt to do what's right now by eating healthy.

Diabetes

Some people still mistakenly assume that diabetes is something you can only suffer from when you're young. Others erroneously believe it's only hereditary. However, diabetes is a disease you can incur anytime and even if you do not like eating sweets a lot. There are other ways for your body's glucose levels to reach abnormal rates, but you can combat them effectively just by eating healthy.

Aside from those mentioned above, eating right can also help lower your risk for various types of cancer and heart diseases. As you can see, healthy eating is the first and best step you can take to enjoying a long, healthy and fulfilling life.

www.ingramcontent.com/pod-product-compliance
Lightning Source LLC
LaVergne TN
LVHW020500080526
838202LV00057B/6071